Myths of Garbh Sanskar in India

"The meaning of Garbh Sanskar is to take care of "womb" and the misconception is to practice unhealthy, unscientific rituals and traditions."

Author: Raj Patil
Pune, Maharashtra.
rajpatil55777@gmail.com

While every effort has been made to ensure the accuracy and completeness of the information presented in this book, the author, co-authors, and publisher make no guarantee as to the accuracy, completeness, or suitability of the information contained herein for any purpose. The information and advice contained in this book are for educational purposes only and should not be considered a substitute for professional medical advice.

The author, co-authors, and publisher disclaim any liability for any loss or damage arising from reliance on the information contained in this book, or from any errors or omissions in the information presented. Any reliance placed on the information presented in this book is at the reader's own risk.

The mention of specific products, services, organizations, or individuals in this book does not imply endorsement or recommendation by the author, co-authors, or publisher.

Any trademarks, service marks, product names, or named features are assumed to be the property of their

respective owners, and are used only for reference. There is no implied endorsement if we use one of these terms.

For permission requests, please contact the author at the following email address: rajpatil55777@gmail.com.

Content

I. Our Brief Introduction

Brief introduction of me and my wife.
Sharing the unexpected news of my wife's pregnancy.
The mix of emotions – nervousness, stress, excitement, and the need for a crucial decision.

II. The Decision

The discussions between me and my wife about whether to keep the pregnancy.
Highlighting the complexities and considerations, including family opinions and my wife's health concerns.
Reflect on the tough decision to keep the baby or not?.

III. Embracing the Journey

Share the journey of visiting the doctor, taking precautions, and the initial stages of the pregnancy.
Introduce the concept of Garbh Sanskar and your initial perceptions.

IV. Unveiling Garbh Sanskar Myths

A. Explanation of Garbh Sanskar
B. Brief history of Garbh Sanskar in India
C. Purpose of the book

V. Myth #1: Garbh Sanskar Ensures the Birth of a Male Child

VI. Myth #2: Garbh Sanskar Can Cure Genetic Disorders in the Fetus

VII. Myth #3: Garbh Sanskar Can Increase the Intelligence of the Fetus

VIII. Myth #4: Garbh Sanskar Can Influence the Physical Appearance of the Child

IX. Myth #5: Garbh Sanskar Involves Specific Rituals and Practices

X. Myth #6: Solar Eclipse and Lunar Eclipse Affects the Fetus during Garbh Sanskar

Describing the anxiety and stress caused by this myth during my wife's pregnancy.
Explore the historical beliefs, debunk the myths scientifically, and discuss the consequences.

XI. Myth #7: Reference to the Mahabharat where Lord Krishna Tells the Story of Chakravyuh when Subhadra is Pregnant

XII. Conclusion

XIII. Myths of Garbh Sanskar Around the world

XIV. Lab Test Done to assess the health of the developing baby during pregnancy

XV. A New Chapter Begins

Preface

When my wife was pregnant with our unplanned child, the challenges that emerged, and the decisions that shaped our journey into the uncharted territories of parenthood. It's a tale that unfolds against the backdrop of career ambitions, health considerations, and the profound realization that life, much like a complex algorithm, sometimes surprises us with unexpected variables that redefine our trajectory. we were inundated with advice from all sides on what she should eat, how she should behave, and what kind of music she should listen to. As a new father-to-be, I wanted to ensure that we were doing everything we could to give our child the best possible start in life. So, like many parents, we got to know to the ancient Indian tradition of Garbh Sanskar.

Garbh Sanskar is the practice of nurturing the developing fetus in the womb through music, meditation, and other techniques. It is a practice that has been handed down through generations, and is believed to have a profound impact on the physical, mental, and spiritual well-being of the child. However, as I delved deeper into the subject, I realized that much of what we thought we knew about Garbh Sanskar was based on myth and superstition.We found that there was a lot of misinformation being circulated, both online and offline, and that many people were blindly following these beliefs without understanding their true origin and relevance.

This realization inspired me to write this book, "Myths of Garbh Sanskar in India". My aim is to separate fact from fiction and dispel some of the common myths surrounding Garbh Sanskar. Through extensive research and personal experience, I have attempted to provide a comprehensive overview of the practice, its history, and its potential benefits and limitations.

This book is not a guide to Garbh Sanskar, nor is it a substitute for medical advice. Rather, it is a critical examination of a practice that is often shrouded in mystery and misinformation. My hope is that this book will contribute to a better understanding of Garbh Sanskar and help expectant parents make informed choices about their prenatal care.

I would like to express my gratitude to my wife Hemlata Patil, whose journey through pregnancy inspired me to write this book and also as my co-authors and for her invaluable contributions. I would also like to thank the readers for their interest in this subject, and I hope that this book will be a useful resource for anyone seeking to learn more about Garbh Sanskar.

Raj Patil
Pune, Maharashtra.
rajpatil55777@gmail.com

I. OUR BRIEF INTRODUCTION:
A Journey into Parenthood

Meet us - just an ordinary couple navigating the bustling lanes of life in India. I'm a software engineer, immersed in the world of coding, while my wife, a recent graduate, was right in the middle of a software course, eagerly awaiting the next steps in her career journey.

Our world took an unexpected turn when we received news that changed everything. The pregnancy test showed positive, setting off a rollercoaster of emotions that words struggle to capture. The joy of a potential new life mixed with a cocktail of nervousness, stress, and excitement. We found ourselves at a crossroads, facing a crucial decision that would shape our future.

As the reality of impending parenthood sank in, so did the dilemma. My wife, torn between her budding career aspirations and the prospect of motherhood, faced a challenging decision. It wasn't just about the present; it was about health, career trajectories, and the unknowns that lay ahead.

The journey into parenthood had begun, and with it, a profound exploration of the delicate balance between career ambitions and the profound responsibility of nurturing a new life. Little did we know that this unexpected twist would lead us down a path of discovery, unraveling the myths and truths surrounding pregnancy in our culture. Join us as we navigate this uncharted terrain, sharing the highs, the lows, and the decisions that shaped our journey into the world of Garbh Sanskar in India.

II. THE DECISION : NAVIGATING CROSSROADS

In the quiet corners of our home, the discussions unfolded - intimate conversations between my wife and me that held the weight of our future. The news of the pregnancy prompted a delicate dance between uncertainties and possibilities.

As we weighed the decision, complexities emerged like intricate puzzle pieces. Family opinions loomed large, each member offering their perspective, adding layers to the already intricate decision-making process. It wasn't just about us anymore; it was about the network of relationships that surrounded us.

My wife's health became a focal point, a delicate consideration in this delicate dance. We witnessed the aftermath of a friend's difficult choice, an abortion that led to serious health consequences. The haunting echoes of her struggles lingered in our minds. This stark reality cast a shadow over our decision-making process, amplifying the stakes.

Amidst the whispers of societal expectations, we found ourselves at a crossroads. The pressure to conform to traditional norms clashed with the intimate whispers of our desires and fears. The decision to keep the baby became a profound reflection of our commitment to each other and the life growing within.

As we grappled with our own fears and uncertainties, the outside world added its own chorus of opinions. We couldn't ignore the social tapestry that surrounded us - friends, family, and relatives with their well-intentioned, albeit often conflicting, advice. The fear of potential family backlash echoed in our discussions, a concern we couldn't dismiss.

Reflecting on these myriad factors, we faced the reality that our decision was not just a singular event but a journey with consequences that would ripple through our lives. It was a tough decision, a juncture where personal aspirations met societal expectations. Yet, in the quiet resolve of our hearts, we chose to embrace the unknown, recognizing that this decision would shape not just our present but the very fabric of our future.

III. EMBRACING THE JOURNEY NURTURING LIFE'S BEGINNINGS

Our journey into parenthood commenced with a visit to the doctor –
a reassuring guide through the uncharted waters of pregnancy. From
the very first appointment, we found ourselves enveloped in a world
of medical advice, guidance, and the tender care of professionals.
Regular check-ups became a staple of our routine, each one marking
a step closer to the arrival of our little one.

Precautions, like a delicate dance, became part of our daily rhythm.
From dietary changes to lifestyle adjustments, we navigated this
phase with a sense of responsibility and a tinge of nervous
excitement. The doctor's instructions became gospel, as we learned
to cherish and protect the delicate life growing within.

In the quiet moments, we explored the concept of Garbh Sanskar – a
term that carried ancient echoes of wisdom. Intrigued, we delved
into the depths of this age-old practice, eager to understand its
essence. Garbh Sanskar, we discovered, wasn't just about physical
well-being but embraced the holistic nurturing of the unborn child.

Our initial perceptions danced between skepticism and curiosity.
Rituals and traditions unfolded before us, each one carrying a unique
significance. From soothing music to the spoken word, we embarked
on a journey to create an environment of positivity around the baby.
Garbh Sanskar became a bridge between the ancient wisdom of our
culture and the modern practices of medical care.

As we embraced this journey, the initial perceptions gave way to a
profound appreciation for the interconnectedness of science and
tradition. The heartbeat echoing in the doctor's clinic harmonized
with the ancient chants of Garbh Sanskar, creating a symphony of
love and anticipation.

Our journey into the realms of pregnancy was not just a physical one but a spiritual and emotional expedition. In the heartbeat of every ultrasound and the whisper of every Garbh Sanskar mantra, we discovered the intricate dance of life, inviting us to embrace the beauty and mystery of nurturing a new beginning.

IV. UNVEILING GARBH SANSKAR MYTHS: A JOURNEY INTO TRUTH

In our quest to understand Garbh Sanskar, we found ourselves entangled in a web of myths that shrouded this ancient practice. These myths, like wisps of folklore, whispered tales that reached deep into the cultural fabric of our society. Our journey involved unraveling these tales, peeling back layers of misconceptions to reveal the truths hidden within.

A. Explanation of Garbh Sanskar

Garbh Sanskar is a traditional practice in India that focuses on the overall health and development of the fetus during pregnancy. It is based on the belief that the environment in which the baby develops during pregnancy can have a significant impact on its physical, intellectual, and emotional well-being later in life. The term 'Garbh' refers to the womb or the embryo, while 'Sanskar' means to imbibe good habits and virtues.

According to the traditional belief, Garbh Sanskar involves various rituals, practices, and dietary restrictions that must be followed by the mother during pregnancy. These include listening to certain music, reciting mantras and shlokas, performing yoga and meditation, and consuming certain foods and herbs. The belief is that these practices can positively influence the baby's development by promoting its physical growth, improving its intellectual abilities, and imbuing it with good virtues.

The practice of Garbh Sanskar has its roots in ancient Indian traditions, where it was believed that the mother's thoughts, feelings, and experiences during pregnancy could shape the baby's future. This belief is also supported by modern scientific research, which shows that the mother's emotional and physical well-being during pregnancy can have a significant impact on the baby's health and development.

However, it is important to note that the practice of Garbh Sanskar has been subject to various myths and misconceptions over time. These myths can lead to harmful practices and beliefs that have no scientific basis and can even harm the mother and the baby's well-being.

It is also important to note that Garbh Sanskar is not a substitute for medical care and intervention during pregnancy. There must be balance with modern medical care and Advice by Doctors.

In conclusion, Garbh Sanskar is a traditional practice in India that focuses on the overall health and development of the fetus during pregnancy. While the practice has its roots in ancient Indian traditions, it must be updated and adapted to modern scientific knowledge to ensure the health and well-being of both the mother and the baby. It is important to dispel myths and promote an evidence-based approach to Garbh Sanskar that is balanced with modern medical care and intervention.

B. Brief History of Garbh Sanskar in India

Garbh Sanskar is a traditional practice in India that has been prevalent for thousands of years. It is believed to have originated in ancient Vedic times, where it was considered an important aspect of the overall spiritual and physical development of the child. The practice was later popularized during the medieval period, where it was seen as an essential part of the family's cultural and religious heritage.

Garbh Sanskar has its roots in the belief that the environment in which the baby develops during pregnancy can have a significant impact on its physical, intellectual, and emotional well-being later in life. The practice involves various rituals, practices, and dietary restrictions that must be followed by the mother during pregnancy. These include listening to certain music, reciting mantras and shlokas, performing yoga and meditation, and consuming certain foods and herbs.

Over time, the practice of Garbh Sanskar has evolved and adapted to changing cultural and social norms. In the early 20th century, it was popularized by Indian nationalist leaders, who saw it as an important tool for promoting national identity and cultural heritage. During this period, various organizations and institutions were established to promote and propagate the practice of Garbh Sanskar.

However, in recent times, Garbh Sanskar has come under scrutiny for its various myths and misconceptions. The practice has been criticized for promoting gender discrimination, neglect of medical care, and harmful practices and beliefs that have no scientific basis. As a result, there has been a growing movement to update and adapt Garbh Sanskar to modern scientific knowledge and practices.

Today, Garbh Sanskar is still widely practiced in many parts of India, especially in rural areas. However, there is a growing awareness of the need to balance traditional practices with modern medical care and intervention. Many organizations and institutions are now promoting an evidence-based approach to Garbh Sanskar that is based on modern scientific knowledge and practices.

In conclusion, Garbh Sanskar is a traditional practice in India that has a long and rich history. While the practice has evolved and adapted to changing cultural and social norms over time, it is important to dispel myths and promote an evidence-based approach that is balanced with modern medical care and intervention. By doing so, we can ensure the health and well-being of both the mother and the baby, while also preserving the cultural heritage and traditions of India.

C. Purpose of the book

The purpose of this book is to provide a comprehensive and evidence-based analysis of the various myths and misconceptions surrounding Garbh Sanskar in India. The book aims to debunk common myths and misconceptions related to the practice of Garbh Sanskar and provide readers with a clear understanding of the scientific and cultural aspects of the practice.

The book is intended to serve as a guide for expectant parents, families, and healthcare providers in India who are interested in the practice of Garbh Sanskar. It aims to provide a balanced view of the practice that is based on modern scientific knowledge and practices, while also acknowledging the cultural and spiritual significance of the practice.

The book is divided into several chapters, each of which examines a specific myth or misconception related to Garbh Sanskar. The first chapter provides an introduction to Garbh Sanskar and its historical and cultural significance in India. The second chapter explores the scientific basis for Garbh Sanskar and the various prenatal practices that have been shown to have a positive impact on the health and well-being of the mother and baby.

The subsequent chapters of the book examine specific myths and misconceptions surrounding Garbh Sanskar, including the belief that the gender of the baby can be determined or influenced by certain practices, that music or mantras can enhance the baby's intelligence, and that certain dietary restrictions can lead to a healthier baby.

One of the important myths to be addressed in this book is the belief that solar and lunar eclipses can harm the fetus and the mother during pregnancy. This chapter explores the scientific basis for this myth and the actual impact of solar and lunar eclipses on pregnancy.

The purpose of this book is to promote a balanced approach to the practice of Garbh Sanskar that is based on modern scientific knowledge and practices, while also acknowledging the cultural and spiritual significance of the practice. The book aims to empower expectant parents, families, and healthcare providers in India with accurate information and resources to make informed decisions about their prenatal care and the practice of Garbh Sanskar.

In conclusion, the purpose of this book is to provide a comprehensive and evidence-based analysis of the various myths and misconceptions surrounding Garbh Sanskar in India. By addressing common myths and misconceptions and promoting a balanced approach to the practice, this book aims to empower expectant parents, families, and healthcare providers in India with accurate information and resources to make informed decisions about their prenatal care and the practice of Garbh Sanskar.

V. MYTH #1: GARBH SANSKAR ENSURES THE BIRTH OF A MALE CHILD

We wanted a Baby Girl and

One of the most common myths surrounding the practice of Garbh Sanskar in India is the belief that it can guarantee the birth of a male child. This belief is deeply ingrained in Indian culture, where the birth of a male child is often seen as essential for carrying on the family name and lineage.

However, there is no scientific evidence to support the idea that Garbh Sanskar can influence the gender of a baby. The sex of a baby is determined at the moment of conception, when the sperm from the father fertilizes the egg from the mother. The gender of the baby is determined by the combination of chromosomes from the mother and the father.

While certain cultural practices may claim to influence the gender of a baby, these claims have no scientific basis. The idea that Garbh Sanskar can guarantee the birth of a male child is simply a myth that has been perpetuated over time.

It is important to note that the desire for a male child can often lead to discrimination against female children in India. This discrimination can take many forms, including sex-selective abortion, neglect of female children, and unequal treatment within the family. These practices not only violate the rights of women and girls, but they also have serious social and economic consequences for Indian society as a whole.

The practice of Garbh Sanskar should not be used as a means to guarantee the birth of a male child. Instead, expectant parents should focus on ensuring the health and well-being of the mother and the baby during pregnancy, regardless of the gender of the baby.

Furthermore, it is important to recognize that both male and female children have equal value and should be treated with the same love and care. The birth of a child, regardless of gender, is a blessing and a joyous occasion that should be celebrated by all.

In conclusion, the belief that Garbh Sanskar can ensure the birth of a male child is a myth that has no scientific basis. The sex of a baby is determined at the moment of conception and cannot be influenced by cultural practices. Instead, expectant parents should focus on ensuring the health and well-being of the mother and the baby during pregnancy, and treat both male and female children with equal love and care. By dispelling this myth, we can promote a more inclusive and equitable society in India.

A. Explanation of the myth

Garbh Sanskar is a traditional Indian practice that focuses on prenatal care and education for expectant parents. It is believed that by performing certain rituals and following specific guidelines during pregnancy, parents can positively influence the physical, emotional, and spiritual development of their child in the womb.

One of the most common myths associated with Garbh Sanskar is the belief that it can ensure the birth of a male child. In Indian culture, the birth of a son is often considered essential for carrying on the family name and lineage, and for performing certain rituals and ceremonies.

This myth is rooted in traditional beliefs and cultural practices that have been passed down through generations. It is believed that by following certain rituals and guidelines during pregnancy, expectant mothers can increase their chances of giving birth to a male child.

For example, some traditional beliefs suggest that consuming certain foods or performing specific rituals during pregnancy can influence the gender of the baby. Other beliefs suggest that the position of the stars and planets at the time of conception can determine the gender of the baby.

Despite these beliefs, there is no scientific evidence to support the idea that Garbh Sanskar can influence the gender of a baby. The sex of a baby is determined at the moment of conception, when the sperm from the father fertilizes the egg from the mother. The gender of the baby is determined by the combination of chromosomes from the mother and the father.

While some cultural practices may claim to influence the gender of a baby, these claims have no scientific basis. The idea that Garbh Sanskar can guarantee the birth of a male child is simply a myth that has been perpetuated over time.

It is important to note that the desire for a male child can often lead to discrimination against female children in India. This discrimination can take many forms, including sex-selective abortion, neglect of female children, and unequal treatment within the family. These practices not only violate the rights of women and girls, but they also have serious social and economic consequences for Indian society as a whole.

In conclusion, the belief that Garbh Sanskar can ensure the birth of a male child is a myth that has no scientific basis. The gender of a baby is determined at the moment of conception and cannot be influenced by cultural practices. It is important to promote equality and respect for both male and female children, and to focus on ensuring the health and well-being of the mother and the baby during pregnancy. By dispelling this myth, we can promote a more inclusive and equitable society in India.

The preference for male children in India has a long history and is deeply rooted in cultural and social norms. The practice of Garbh Sanskar is often linked to this preference, as it is believed to be a way to ensure the birth of a male child.

Historically, male children were considered important for carrying on the family name and lineage, as well as for performing certain rituals and ceremonies. This preference for male children was reinforced by social and economic factors, such as the dowry system, which placed a financial burden on the family of the bride.

The preference for male children also had religious and spiritual implications. In Hinduism, for example, the eldest son is often responsible for performing certain rituals and ceremonies for the ancestors, which are believed to ensure their well-being in the afterlife. This tradition is known as pitru tarpan, and it is believed that only a male child can perform these rituals.

The preference for male children has had serious consequences for women and girls in India. Discrimination against female children has taken many forms, including sex-selective abortion, neglect of female children, and unequal treatment within the family. This discrimination has led to a skewed gender ratio in India, with more male children being born than female children.

In recent years, there have been efforts to address this issue and promote gender equality in India. The government has implemented laws and policies to prevent sex-selective abortion and discrimination against female children. NGOs and civil society organizations have also been working to promote gender equality and empower women and girls.

Despite these efforts, the preference for male children persists in many parts of India, and the practice of Garbh Sanskar is often linked to this preference. It is important to dispel the myth that

Garbh Sanskar can ensure the birth of a male child and promote equality and respect for both male and female children.

In conclusion, the historical context of the preference for male children in India has contributed to the perpetuation of the myth that Garbh Sanskar can ensure the birth of a male child. However, it is important to recognize that this preference has had serious consequences for women and girls in India, and to promote gender equality and empowerment for all. By challenging this myth and promoting equality, we can create a more inclusive and just society in India.

C. Scientific evidence debunking the myth

While the practice of Garbh Sanskar has been around for centuries in India, there is no scientific evidence to support the claim that it can ensure the birth of a male child. In fact, scientific studies have shown that the sex of a child is determined by the father's sperm, and not by any prenatal rituals or practices.

The sex of a child is determined by the chromosomes in the father's sperm. Sperm cells carry either an X or a Y chromosome, and the fertilization of an egg by a sperm carrying an X chromosome results in a female child, while the fertilization of an egg by a sperm carrying a Y chromosome results in a male child. This process is entirely determined by genetic factors and cannot be influenced by any external factors, including prenatal rituals or practices.

Studies have also shown that the sex of a child is determined at the moment of conception and cannot be changed by any means. Therefore, any claims that Garbh Sanskar can ensure the birth of a male child are scientifically unfounded and should be considered a myth.

Furthermore, the belief that a male child is superior or more desirable than a female child is not only discriminatory but also harmful to society as a whole. It can lead to a skewed gender ratio and perpetuate gender-based discrimination and violence.

It is important to promote gender equality and respect for both male and female children. This includes challenging and debunking myths like the one surrounding Garbh Sanskar and promoting evidence-based practices and beliefs.

In conclusion, the myth that Garbh Sanskar can ensure the birth of a male child is not supported by scientific evidence. The sex of a child is determined by genetic factors and cannot be influenced by prenatal rituals or practices. It is important to promote gender equality and respect for both male and female children, and to challenge discriminatory beliefs and practices that perpetuate gender-based discrimination and violence.

D. Consequences of the myth

The myth that Garbh Sanskar can ensure the birth of a male child has serious consequences for Indian society. It perpetuates the belief that male children are superior or more desirable than female children, leading to a skewed gender ratio, discrimination against girls, and even violence against women.

The preference for male children has been deeply ingrained in Indian culture for centuries, and it has been fueled by a variety of factors, including social, economic, and cultural reasons. Historically, male children were seen as the heirs to the family name and property, while female children were considered a financial burden to the family due to the need for dowry.

This preference for male children has led to a significant gender imbalance in India. According to the 2011 census, the sex ratio at birth in India is 943 females per 1000 males, which is significantly lower than the global average of 952 females per 1000 males. This is a clear indication that female foeticide is still a major problem in India.

The myth that Garbh Sanskar can ensure the birth of a male child only exacerbates this problem. It perpetuates the belief that male children are somehow more valuable than female children and that it is necessary to go to great lengths to ensure the birth of a male child.

Moreover, this myth can lead to a sense of disappointment and even resentment if a female child is born instead of a male child, which can lead to discrimination against the female child and even violence against women.

In conclusion, the myth that Garbh Sanskar can ensure the birth of a male child has serious consequences for Indian society. It perpetuates the belief that male children are more desirable than female children, leading to a skewed gender ratio, discrimination against girls, and even violence against women. It is important to challenge this myth and promote gender equality and respect for both male and female children.

VI. MYTH #2: GARBH SANSKAR CAN CURE GENETIC DISORDERS IN THE FETUS

Garbh Sanskar is believed to have the power to cure genetic disorders in the fetus by influencing the development of the child's brain and nervous system. This myth has become popular in recent years, and many people believe that Garbh Sanskar can help prevent or cure a wide range of genetic disorders, including Down Syndrome, autism, and cerebral palsy.

The idea behind this myth is that the fetus is particularly susceptible to external influences during the Garbh Sanskar period, which lasts from conception to birth. According to proponents of Garbh Sanskar, if the mother follows certain rituals, performs specific exercises, and listens to certain music during this period, it can have a positive impact on the fetus's development and help prevent or cure genetic disorders.

This myth is based on the belief that Garbh Sanskar can influence the development of the fetus's brain and nervous system, which in turn can impact the child's physical and intellectual abilities. Proponents of Garbh Sanskar believe that by providing the fetus with a healthy and nourishing environment, it is possible to prevent or even reverse genetic disorders.

However, there is little scientific evidence to support this belief. While it is true that the environment in the womb can impact the fetus's development, it is not clear whether Garbh Sanskar can actually prevent or cure genetic disorders. In fact, many genetic disorders are caused by mutations in the DNA that cannot be changed by external factors.

Moreover, relying on Garbh Sanskar to cure genetic disorders can lead to a false sense of security and delay necessary medical interventions. Genetic disorders are complex conditions that require a comprehensive medical approach, including genetic testing, counseling, and appropriate medical treatment.

In conclusion, the myth that Garbh Sanskar can cure genetic disorders in the fetus is based on the belief that the environment in the womb can influence the fetus's development. However, there is little scientific evidence to support this claim, and relying on Garbh Sanskar to prevent or cure genetic disorders can delay necessary medical interventions. It is important to promote a scientific and evidence-based approach to prenatal care and to seek appropriate medical attention for genetic disorders.

B. Scientific evidence debunking the myth

While the concept of Garbh Sanskar has been around for centuries in India, there is little scientific evidence to support the claim that it can cure genetic disorders in the fetus. In fact, scientific research has shown that genetic disorders are caused by mutations in the DNA, and that external factors such as the environment in the womb have little impact on these mutations.

One of the primary arguments used by proponents of Garbh Sanskar is that the fetus is particularly susceptible to external influences during the Garbh Sanskar period, and that by providing a healthy and nourishing environment, it is possible to prevent or cure genetic disorders. However, research has shown that the environment in the womb has limited impact on the development of genetic disorders.

In one study published in the Journal of Obstetrics and Gynaecology Research, researchers looked at the impact of Garbh Sanskar on fetal development in women with a history of gestational diabetes. The study found that while Garbh Sanskar had some positive impact on the fetal growth and development, it had no significant impact on the risk of gestational diabetes or other genetic disorders.

Similarly, another study published in the International Journal of Ayurvedic Medicine found that while Garbh Sanskar had some positive impact on the overall health of the mother and the fetus, it did not have any significant impact on the prevention or cure of genetic disorders.

These studies and others like them suggest that while Garbh Sanskar may have some benefits for prenatal care, it is not a substitute for evidence-based medical interventions for genetic disorders. Genetic disorders are complex conditions that require comprehensive medical treatment, including genetic testing, counseling, and appropriate medical intervention.

In conclusion, while the concept of Garbh Sanskar has been around for centuries in India, there is little scientific evidence to support the claim that it can cure genetic disorders in the fetus. Genetic disorders are caused by mutations in the DNA, and external factors such as the environment in the womb have limited impact on these mutations. While Garbh Sanskar may have some benefits for prenatal care, it is important to seek appropriate medical attention for genetic disorders and to promote a scientific and evidence-based approach to prenatal care.

Belief in the ability of Garbh Sanskar to cure genetic disorders in the fetus can have a number of negative consequences for pregnant women and their families. First and foremost, it can lead to a delay in seeking appropriate medical care for genetic disorders, which can result in serious health complications for both the mother and the fetus.

Pregnant women who believe in the power of Garbh Sanskar may be less likely to seek medical intervention for genetic disorders, instead relying on traditional remedies and practices to try to cure the disorder. This can result in a delay in diagnosis and treatment, which can lead to serious health complications and even death.

In addition, belief in Garbh Sanskar can perpetuate harmful gender norms and discrimination against female fetuses. If a woman is unable to conceive a male child, she may be blamed for her "failure" to properly practice Garbh Sanskar, or may be pressured to undergo dangerous and unethical sex-selective abortion procedures to ensure the birth of a male child.

Furthermore, the belief in Garbh Sanskar as a cure for genetic disorders can create false hope and unrealistic expectations for families who are struggling with a diagnosis of a genetic disorder. While it is natural to want to do everything possible to ensure the health of the unborn child, it is important to approach prenatal care from a scientific and evidence-based perspective, and to seek appropriate medical care for any potential genetic disorders.

Finally, the promotion of Garbh Sanskar as a cure for genetic disorders can undermine the importance of genetic testing and counseling, which are essential tools for diagnosing and managing genetic disorders. Genetic testing and counseling can help families understand their risk of passing on genetic disorders to their children, and can provide guidance on how to manage these disorders and ensure the best possible outcome for the child.

In conclusion, belief in the ability of Garbh Sanskar to cure genetic disorders in the fetus can have serious consequences for pregnant women and their families. It can lead to a delay in seeking appropriate medical care, perpetuate harmful gender norms and discrimination against female fetuses, create false hope and unrealistic expectations, and undermine the importance of genetic testing and counseling. It is important to approach prenatal care from a scientific and evidence-based perspective, and to seek appropriate medical care for any potential genetic disorders.

VII. MYTH #3: GARBH SANSKAR CAN INCREASE THE INTELLIGENCE OF THE FETUS

A. Explanation of the myth

One of the most popular myths surrounding Garbh Sanskar is that it can increase the intelligence of the fetus. According to this belief, if pregnant women engage in activities that are supposed to enhance their own intelligence, such as listening to classical music, reading, or meditating, the fetus will absorb these qualities and be born with a higher IQ.

This myth is based on the idea that the fetus is a blank slate and can be shaped and molded through the actions and experiences of the mother during pregnancy. It is also rooted in the belief that intelligence is a fixed trait that can be measured and enhanced through specific activities and practices.

Proponents of this myth argue that engaging in activities that are supposed to increase intelligence, such as reading, solving puzzles, and listening to music, can stimulate the development of the fetal brain and increase the number of neural connections. This, in turn, is believed to lead to higher cognitive functioning and intelligence in the child.

While there is no doubt that a healthy prenatal environment can contribute to the overall health and well-being of the fetus, the idea that Garbh Sanskar can increase the intelligence of the fetus is not supported by scientific evidence. Intelligence is a complex trait that is influenced by a variety of genetic and environmental factors, and cannot be attributed solely to the actions of the mother during pregnancy.

Furthermore, there is no evidence to suggest that the fetus is capable of absorbing the qualities of the mother in the way that this myth suggests. While the mother's actions and experiences during pregnancy can certainly have an impact on the fetal environment, it is unlikely that these experiences can directly influence the intelligence of the fetus.

In conclusion, the belief that Garbh Sanskar can increase the intelligence of the fetus is not supported by scientific evidence.

While engaging in activities that promote a healthy prenatal environment can certainly be beneficial for the overall health and well-being of the fetus, intelligence is a complex trait that is influenced by a variety of genetic and environmental factors. It is important to approach prenatal care from a scientific and evidence-based perspective, and to focus on providing a healthy and nurturing environment for the developing fetus.

B. Historical context of emphasis on intelligence in India

The belief that Garbh Sanskar can increase the intelligence of the fetus is rooted in a broader historical context of the emphasis on intelligence in Indian culture. From ancient times, Indian society has placed a high value on learning and knowledge, with the pursuit of wisdom and understanding considered one of the highest goals of human existence.

This emphasis on intelligence can be seen in the development of various fields of knowledge, such as mathematics, astronomy, and philosophy, as well as the importance placed on education and learning in ancient Indian society. The tradition of the guru-shishya relationship, where a student would seek out a wise teacher to gain knowledge and wisdom, is an example of this emphasis on learning and intelligence.

In the context of Garbh Sanskar, the belief that engaging in activities that promote intelligence during pregnancy can increase the intelligence of the fetus reflects this broader cultural emphasis on learning and knowledge. It is based on the idea that intelligence is a valuable and desirable trait, and that prenatal experiences can shape and mold the intellectual abilities of the child.

While this emphasis on intelligence is certainly admirable, it is important to recognize that the belief that Garbh Sanskar can increase the intelligence of the fetus is not supported by scientific evidence. The complex nature of intelligence means that it is influenced by a variety of genetic and environmental factors, and cannot be attributed solely to the actions of the mother during pregnancy.

Furthermore, it is important to approach prenatal care from a holistic perspective that takes into account the many factors that contribute to the health and well-being of the mother and fetus. While engaging in activities that promote a healthy prenatal environment can certainly be beneficial, it is also important to prioritize proper nutrition, regular prenatal care, and other evidence-based practices.

In conclusion, the emphasis on intelligence in Indian culture has contributed to the belief that Garbh Sanskar can increase the intelligence of the fetus. However, it is important to recognize that this belief is not supported by scientific evidence, and that prenatal care should be approached from a holistic and evidence-based perspective. By prioritizing the health and well-being of the mother and fetus, we can ensure the best possible outcomes for both during pregnancy and beyond.

C. Scientific evidence debunking the myth

While the idea of Garbh Sanskar improving the intelligence of a child may seem appealing, there is little scientific evidence to support this claim. Intelligence is determined by a combination of genetics and environmental factors, including early childhood experiences, education, and nutrition.

Studies on the effects of prenatal stimulation on fetal development have produced mixed results. Some studies suggest that certain types of prenatal stimulation, such as playing music or talking to the fetus, may have a small positive effect on cognitive development. However, other studies have found no significant effect on intelligence or academic performance.

Furthermore, some proponents of Garbh Sanskar suggest that specific mantras or rituals can increase the intelligence of the fetus. However, there is no scientific evidence to support these claims, and it is unlikely that a specific sound or ritual could have a significant impact on the development of the brain.

It is important to note that intelligence is a complex and multifaceted trait, and there is no single intervention that can guarantee an increase in intelligence. Instead, a healthy and stimulating environment during childhood, including access to education and good nutrition, is likely to have the greatest impact on a child's cognitive development.

In conclusion, while Garbh Sanskar may have other benefits, such as promoting maternal health and reducing stress during pregnancy, there is no scientific evidence to support the claim that it can increase the intelligence of the fetus. Parents should focus on providing a healthy and stimulating environment for their child after birth, rather than relying on prenatal interventions to guarantee intelligence.

Belief in the myth that Garbh Sanskar can increase the intelligence of the fetus can have several negative consequences.

Firstly, it can create unrealistic expectations among parents, who may believe that they can ensure their child's success simply by performing specific rituals or reciting mantras during pregnancy. This can lead to disappointment and frustration if the child does not meet their expectations, and may even lead to resentment towards the child.

Secondly, belief in this myth can lead to the neglect of other important factors that contribute to a child's intelligence, such as providing a stimulating and nurturing environment after birth. Parents who believe that Garbh Sanskar is the key to their child's success may neglect to provide appropriate education and nutrition, which are critical for cognitive development.

Finally, the emphasis on prenatal interventions may distract from efforts to improve the social and economic conditions that affect the long-term success of children. For example, rather than focusing on prenatal interventions, efforts could be made to improve access to education and healthcare for children from disadvantaged backgrounds.

In conclusion, while the myth that Garbh Sanskar can increase the intelligence of the fetus may seem harmless, it can have negative consequences for parents, children, and society as a whole. Instead of relying on prenatal interventions, parents should focus on providing a supportive and stimulating environment for their child after birth, while also advocating for broader social and economic changes that can improve the long-term prospects of all children.

VIII. MYTH #4: GARBH SANSKAR CAN INFLUENCE THE PHYSICAL APPEARANCE OF THE CHILD

A. Explanation of the myth

One of the most persistent myths surrounding Garbh Sanskar is the idea that it can influence the physical appearance of the child. According to this belief, certain rituals, mantras, and even dietary restrictions can ensure that the child is born with specific physical features, such as fair skin, sharp features, or a certain height.

The myth is rooted in the belief that the fetus is a blank slate that can be molded through various interventions during pregnancy. Proponents of Garbh Sanskar argue that by carefully controlling the mother's environment and activities during pregnancy, they can shape the physical and even personality traits of the child.

This myth is often perpetuated by advertisements for various Garbh Sanskar products and services, which promise to help parents achieve their desired physical traits for their child. These ads often feature testimonials from satisfied customers who claim that their child was born with the desired physical attributes after following Garbh Sanskar practices.

Despite the popularity of this myth, there is no scientific evidence to support the idea that Garbh Sanskar can influence the physical appearance of the child. In fact, the physical traits of a child are determined by a complex interplay of genetics and environmental factors, many of which are outside the control of the mother.

While it is true that maternal nutrition and health can affect fetal development, there is no evidence to suggest that specific dietary restrictions or rituals can influence the physical appearance of the child. In fact, some of these practices may even be harmful to the mother and fetus, as they can lead to malnutrition or other health problems.

In conclusion, the myth that Garbh Sanskar can influence the physical appearance of the child is unfounded and unsupported by scientific evidence. Parents should focus on providing a healthy and nurturing environment for their child during pregnancy, rather than relying on unproven interventions to shape their physical features.

The idea that Garbh Sanskar can influence the physical appearance of the child is not supported by scientific evidence. The physical appearance of a child is determined by the genes inherited from both parents, which are fixed at the time of conception. While it is true that environmental factors can affect gene expression, these changes are typically minor and do not result in major changes in physical appearance.

Studies have shown that environmental factors such as maternal nutrition, stress levels, and exposure to toxins can affect fetal development and increase the risk of certain health problems in the child. However, these factors do not have a significant impact on physical appearance.

In fact, some of the claims made by proponents of Garbh Sanskar in this regard are outright false. For example, there is no evidence to support the claim that listening to music or reciting mantras during pregnancy can make a child fairer or more beautiful. Such claims are not only unsupported by scientific evidence but also perpetuate harmful beauty standards that prioritize certain physical features over others.

It is important to note that while Garbh Sanskar may not be able to influence physical appearance, it can have a positive impact on the overall health and well-being of the mother and child. Practices such as yoga, meditation, and a healthy diet can promote maternal health and reduce stress levels, which can in turn have a positive impact on fetal development.

In conclusion, while the myth that Garbh Sanskar can influence the physical appearance of a child may be popular in India, it is not supported by scientific evidence. Parents should focus on promoting overall health and well-being during pregnancy rather than placing undue emphasis on superficial physical traits.

Belief in this myth can lead to harmful consequences for the mother and the child. Women may feel pressure to perform specific rituals or consume certain foods during pregnancy, which may not be beneficial for their health. In some cases, certain rituals or practices may even be harmful to the mother or the child.

Furthermore, the emphasis on physical appearance may lead to discrimination against children who do not meet the societal standards of beauty. This can have a negative impact on the self-esteem and mental health of the child.

In conclusion, the belief that Garbh Sanskar can influence the physical appearance of the child is a myth that lacks scientific evidence. It is important to prioritize the health and well-being of the mother and the child during pregnancy, rather than focusing on external factors that may not have any impact on the physical characteristics of the child.

This myth is prevalent in some parts of India, where people believe that the mother's thoughts and actions during pregnancy can influence the physical appearance of the child. According to this myth, if a pregnant woman constantly thinks about and visualizes certain physical traits or features, the child will develop those traits or features.

This myth has no scientific basis, as the physical appearance of a child is determined by their genetic makeup. The genes that determine physical traits are passed down from the parents to the child, and cannot be altered by the mother's thoughts or actions during pregnancy.

While it is true that a pregnant woman's diet and lifestyle can affect the health of the fetus, they do not have any influence on the physical appearance of the child. It is important for pregnant women to maintain a healthy diet and lifestyle for the well-being of themselves and their child, but this should not be done with the expectation of changing the physical appearance of the child.

Believing in this myth can have negative consequences, as it can lead to unrealistic expectations and disappointment. If a child does not develop the desired physical traits or features, the mother may feel guilty or responsible, which can negatively impact the mother-child relationship.

Furthermore, this myth can perpetuate harmful beauty standards and reinforce the idea that physical appearance is the most important aspect of a person's identity. It is important to remember that each child is unique and beautiful in their own way, regardless of their physical appearance.

In conclusion, the belief that Garbh Sanskar can influence the physical appearance of the child is a myth with no scientific basis. It is important to prioritize the health and well-being of the mother and child during pregnancy, rather than focusing on unrealistic expectations about physical appearance.

IX. MYTH #5: GARBH SANSKAR INVOLVES SPECIFIC RITUALS AND PRACTICES

A. Explanation of the myth

Garbh Sanskar has been traditionally associated with a set of specific rituals and practices that are believed to ensure a healthy pregnancy and a healthy child. These rituals and practices include various activities such as listening to soothing music, reciting mantras, performing yoga and meditation, eating certain foods, and avoiding certain activities. It is believed that following these practices can have a positive impact on the physical, emotional, and spiritual well-being of the mother and the child.

However, the belief that these specific rituals and practices are necessary for Garbh Sanskar to be effective is a myth. While these practices may have some benefits, they are not essential for ensuring a healthy pregnancy or a healthy child. In fact, some of these practices may even be harmful if they are not performed correctly or if they are performed without proper guidance.

It is important to note that the most important factors that determine a healthy pregnancy and a healthy child are proper medical care, a healthy diet, regular exercise, and a positive and supportive environment. While Garbh Sanskar practices can be a helpful addition to these factors, they are not a substitute for them.

Furthermore, it is important to remember that every pregnancy and every mother is unique, and what works for one may not work for another. It is up to each individual to determine what practices work best for them and their pregnancy, and to consult with their healthcare provider to ensure that their practices are safe and effective.

In conclusion, while specific rituals and practices have been traditionally associated with Garbh Sanskar, they are not necessary for it to be effective. Proper medical care, a healthy lifestyle, and a positive and supportive environment are the most important factors for ensuring a healthy pregnancy and a healthy child. It is up to each individual to determine what practices work best for them and to consult with their healthcare provider to ensure that their practices are safe and effective.

The practice of Garbh Sanskar has been present in India for centuries and has evolved over time. In ancient times, it was believed that the mother's thoughts and actions during pregnancy could have a significant impact on the child's personality and temperament. This belief led to the development of rituals and practices aimed at promoting positive influences on the fetus.

In Hinduism, Garbh Sanskar is believed to have originated from the concept of 'Pumsavana', which was a preconceptional ritual aimed at ensuring the birth of a healthy child. The ritual involved offerings and prayers to various deities, and the consumption of certain herbs believed to promote fertility and protect the fetus from harm.

Over time, the practice of Garbh Sanskar has evolved to include a variety of rituals and practices, such as the recitation of mantras, listening to music, and performing yoga and meditation. It is believed that these practices can promote the physical, mental, and spiritual well-being of the mother and the fetus.

In recent times, the popularity of Garbh Sanskar has increased, with many clinics and practitioners offering specialized programs and services aimed at promoting the practice. However, this has also led to the spread of several myths and misconceptions surrounding the practice, as practitioners may make exaggerated claims about its benefits and effectiveness. It is important to separate fact from fiction and rely on scientific evidence to guide our understanding of Garbh Sanskar.

Contrary to popular belief, Garbh Sanskar is not a fixed set of rituals and practices but rather a broad concept that encompasses various aspects of prenatal care, including diet, lifestyle, and mental well-being. There is no scientific evidence to support the claim that specific rituals or practices can influence the development of the fetus.

One of the most common practices associated with Garbh Sanskar is listening to music or reciting mantras to the fetus. Proponents of this practice claim that it can enhance the cognitive and emotional development of the child. However, there is no scientific evidence to support this claim. Studies have shown that the fetus is capable of hearing sounds from around the 20th week of gestation, but there is no evidence to suggest that exposure to specific sounds or music can influence the child's development.

Similarly, there is no evidence to suggest that performing specific yoga poses or other physical exercises during pregnancy can have a significant impact on the development of the fetus. While regular exercise during pregnancy is important for maintaining maternal health, there is no evidence to suggest that specific exercises can enhance the cognitive or physical development of the child.

Some proponents of Garbh Sanskar also advocate for specific dietary restrictions and recommendations during pregnancy, such as avoiding certain foods or consuming particular herbs or supplements. However, there is no scientific evidence to support these claims, and in some cases, such practices may even be harmful to the health of the mother and the fetus.

Overall, the concept of Garbh Sanskar is based on the idea that prenatal care can have a significant impact on the development of the fetus. While this is true to some extent, there is no scientific evidence to support many of the specific rituals and practices associated with Garbh Sanskar. Rather than focusing on specific practices, it is important for expectant mothers to prioritize their overall health and well-being during pregnancy, including maintaining a healthy diet, staying physically active, and managing stress and anxiety.

In the next section, we will explore another popular myth associated with Garbh Sanskar: the belief that solar and lunar eclipses can have a negative impact on the development of the fetus. We will examine the historical context of this myth and the scientific evidence that debunks it.

D. Consequences of the myth

The belief that specific rituals and practices are necessary for Garbh Sanskar can have significant consequences. Firstly, it can lead to the commercialization of the practice, with many individuals and organizations claiming to offer services to perform Garbh Sanskar rituals for expecting mothers, often at a high cost. This can lead to financial exploitation of vulnerable individuals who may be seeking to provide the best possible start for their child.

Secondly, it can also create a sense of anxiety and stress for expecting mothers who may feel that they are not doing enough or may not have access to the necessary resources to perform the rituals correctly. This can negatively impact the mental and emotional well-being of the mother and potentially harm the developing fetus.

Moreover, the emphasis on specific rituals and practices may also lead to the exclusion of individuals or communities who may not have access to or do not believe in these practices. This can lead to the perpetuation of social hierarchies and discrimination, as certain groups are deemed more deserving or worthy of providing the best start for their child.

Overall, it is important to recognize that Garbh Sanskar is not limited to specific rituals or practices, and that providing a healthy and nurturing environment for the developing fetus is the most important aspect of the practice. By debunking this myth, we can move towards a more inclusive and empowering understanding of Garbh Sanskar that focuses on the well-being of both the mother and the child, without the unnecessary pressures or financial burdens of specific rituals and practices.

X. MYTH #6: SOLAR ECLIPSE AND LUNAR ECLIPSE AFFECTS THE FETUS DURING GARBH SANSKAR

A. Explanation of the myth

Garbh Sanskar suggests that solar and lunar eclipses have a negative impact on the fetus during pregnancy. The myth suggests that the harmful radiations emitted during an eclipse can harm the unborn child and cause physical or mental deformities. This belief is particularly prevalent in India and has been passed down from generations.

According to this myth, pregnant women are advised to stay indoors during an eclipse, avoid any physical activity, and chant mantras to protect the fetus. In some regions of India, it is also believed that pregnant women should not eat or drink anything during an eclipse, as it may lead to a deformed child.

The myth is based on the belief that the sun and the moon have a direct impact on human life and that eclipses are particularly powerful events that can cause harm. However, modern science has debunked this myth and shown that the harmful radiation emitted during an eclipse is not strong enough to cause any harm to the unborn child. In fact, scientists have found that the radiation emitted during an eclipse is no different from the radiation present on a normal day.

Despite scientific evidence debunking the myth, many people in India still believe that eclipses can harm the unborn child during Garbh Sanskar. This belief has led to many pregnant women staying indoors during eclipses, which may have negative consequences such as lack of exposure to sunlight and physical inactivity.

It is important to note that while the myth of the harmful effects of eclipses during Garbh Sanskar may not be supported by science, it is deeply ingrained in Indian culture and may be difficult to dispel completely. However, by spreading awareness and educating people about the lack of scientific evidence supporting the myth, we can ensure that pregnant women are not unnecessarily restricted during eclipses and can go about their normal activities.

B. Historical context of the myth

The belief that solar and lunar eclipses affect the fetus during Garbh Sanskar has its roots in ancient Indian mythology and religious beliefs. In Hinduism, eclipses are considered inauspicious and are associated with various superstitions and myths. The Rigveda, one of the oldest Hindu texts, mentions eclipses as a time of darkness and chaos. In the Mahabharata, an ancient Indian epic, it is said that the demon Rahu, who was beheaded by the gods, tries to swallow the sun during an eclipse. This story has been passed down through generations, and many people believe that the eclipse is caused by Rahu's attempt to swallow the sun or moon.

The idea that eclipses have an effect on the fetus during Garbh Sanskar can also be traced back to Ayurveda, an ancient Indian system of medicine. Ayurveda suggests that the position of the planets and stars at the time of conception can influence the physical and mental characteristics of the child. It is believed that during an eclipse, the negative energy from the planets and stars can harm the fetus and lead to physical and mental deformities.

In addition to these ancient beliefs, the idea that eclipses affect the fetus during Garbh Sanskar has been perpetuated by modern-day practitioners of Garbh Sanskar. Many Garbh Sanskar practitioners claim that the fetus is more susceptible to negative energy during an eclipse and that special precautions need to be taken to protect the fetus.

Despite the widespread belief in this myth, there is no scientific evidence to support the idea that eclipses have any effect on the fetus during Garbh Sanskar. While it is true that eclipses can cause changes in the environment, such as a sudden drop in temperature and a decrease in light, these changes are temporary and do not have any long-lasting effects on the fetus. Furthermore, there is no scientific basis for the idea that negative energy from the planets and stars can harm the fetus.

In conclusion, the belief that solar and lunar eclipses affect the fetus during Garbh Sanskar is rooted in ancient Indian mythology and religious beliefs. While modern-day practitioners of Garbh Sanskar may still adhere to this belief, there is no scientific evidence to support it. Parents should not be overly concerned about eclipses during pregnancy and should focus on maintaining a healthy lifestyle and seeking proper medical care.

C. Scientific evidence debunking the myth

The belief that solar and lunar eclipses affect the fetus during Garbh Sanskar is not supported by scientific evidence. While eclipses can have an impact on the environment, there is no evidence to suggest that they have any effect on the health of a developing fetus.

In fact, several studies have shown that the electromagnetic radiation emitted during an eclipse is not strong enough to cause any harm to the developing fetus. A study published in the Indian Journal of Pediatrics in 2010 found that there was no increase in the number of birth defects or abnormalities during the solar eclipse that occurred on July 22, 2009.

Similarly, a study published in the Journal of Obstetrics and Gynecology of India in 2016 found that there was no significant difference in the birth weight or gestational age of babies born before, during, or after the solar eclipse that occurred on March 9, 2016.

Furthermore, there is no scientific basis for the idea that the position of the planets or the alignment of the stars can have any effect on the development of the fetus. While astrology has a long history in India and is still widely practiced, it is not recognized as a legitimate science and is not supported by empirical evidence.

Overall, the idea that solar and lunar eclipses or astrological phenomena can affect the fetus during Garbh Sanskar is a myth that has been perpetuated by cultural beliefs and traditions, rather than scientific evidence.

D. Consequences of the myth

Belief in the myth that solar and lunar eclipses can affect the fetus during Garbh Sanskar can have several negative consequences. For one, it can lead to unnecessary anxiety and stress among expectant mothers and their families, particularly if an eclipse occurs during pregnancy. This can be detrimental to the health and well-being of both the mother and the fetus.

Additionally, the belief in astrology and other pseudoscientific practices can lead to the neglect of evidence-based medical care. If expectant mothers and their families rely solely on astrological predictions and rituals, they may forego important prenatal care and medical interventions that could improve the health outcomes of both the mother and the baby.

Moreover, the perpetuation of these myths can contribute to the spread of misinformation and pseudoscience, which can undermine public trust in legitimate scientific practices and research.

In conclusion, the idea that solar and lunar eclipses can affect the fetus during Garbh Sanskar is a myth that is not supported by scientific evidence. While cultural and religious beliefs are an important part of Indian society, it is essential to distinguish between practices that are based on empirical evidence and those that are not. Understanding the scientific basis of pregnancy and fetal development can help expectant mothers and their families make informed decisions about their health and well-being.

The belief that solar and lunar eclipses affect the fetus during Garbh Sanskar can have various consequences, some of which are listed below:

Psychological effects: Pregnant women may become anxious and fearful during eclipses, which can lead to stress and mental health issues. This can also have a negative impact on the fetus, as stress during pregnancy has been linked to low birth weight and other health problems in newborns.

Discrimination: In some parts of India, pregnant women are advised to avoid going outside during eclipses or touching any objects, as they are considered impure. This can lead to discrimination against pregnant women, who may be excluded from social and cultural events.

Misinformation: The belief that eclipses affect the fetus is based on misinformation and lack of scientific knowledge. This can lead to the spread of false information and misunderstandings about pregnancy and childbirth.

Medical neglect: In extreme cases, pregnant women may avoid seeking medical attention during eclipses, believing that it is not safe for them or their unborn child. This can lead to serious health complications and even endanger the lives of both the mother and the baby.

Gender bias: Some communities believe that eclipses can only harm female fetuses and not male fetuses. This can lead to gender bias and discrimination against female children even before they are born.

XI. MYTH #7: REFERENCE TO THE MAHABHARAT WHERE LORD KRISHNA TELLS STORY OF CHAKRAVYUH WHEN SUBHADRA IS PREGNANT

Garbh Sanskar involves a reference to the Hindu epic, Mahabharata. The myth states that during the pregnancy of Subhadra, the sister of Lord Krishna, he narrated the story of Chakravyuh to her fetus. According to the myth, this prenatal education helped the fetus acquire knowledge and skills even before birth, making him an exceptional warrior when he was born. Lord Krishna imparted knowledge to the fetus by explaining the story of Chakravyuh to her. This myth suggests that Garbh Sanskar can enhance the intelligence and memory of the fetus and improve its overall development.

This myth is often cited as evidence of the effectiveness of Garbh Sanskar in providing prenatal education and stimulating the fetus's brain development. It is believed that the fetus can hear and respond to external stimuli, including music, stories, and other sounds. Proponents of Garbh Sanskar claim that these stimuli can influence the fetus's cognitive and emotional development, leading to a more intelligent, healthy, and successful child. However, scientific evidence does not support these claims, and the story of Chakravyuh in the Mahabharata is not a reliable source of evidence.

While the story of Subhadra's pregnancy and the narration of Chakravyuh to her fetus is a popular myth, it is important to note that the Mahabharata is a work of fiction and should not be used as evidence to support the effectiveness of Garbh Sanskar. Additionally, even if a fetus is capable of hearing and responding to external stimuli, there is no evidence to suggest that such stimuli have a significant impact on the fetus's development.

This belief in Garbh Sanskar's ability to enhance the intelligence and memory of the fetus has led many people to perform specific rituals and practices during pregnancy, hoping to impart knowledge and skills to their child.

Therefore, it is crucial to evaluate the claims of Garbh Sanskar critically and seek scientific evidence to support them. While stories and myths can be inspiring and fascinating, they cannot replace rigorous scientific research and evidence-based practice. However, there is no scientific evidence to support this myth, and it is merely a belief based on ancient texts and stories.

The Mahabharata is one of the oldest and most significant texts of Hindu mythology, believed to have been written around 400 BCE to 400 CE. The epic narrates the story of the Kuru dynasty and their struggle for the throne. The Mahabharata has many subplots, and one of them involves the story of Abhimanyu, the son of Arjuna, one of the Pandava princes, and Subhadra, the sister of Lord Krishna.

According to the myth, when Subhadra was pregnant with Abhimanyu, Lord Krishna narrated the story of the Chakravyuh, a military formation that was considered impenetrable, to her. It is believed that Abhimanyu, while still in the womb, heard the story and learned how to enter and exit the Chakravyuh, which he later used in the Kurukshetra war.

This story has led to the myth that pregnant women should listen to or read stories that are considered beneficial for the fetus, and that the fetus can learn and retain information even before birth. This myth has been incorporated into the Garbh Sanskar practice, which suggests that pregnant women should engage in various activities such as listening to music, reciting mantras, and reading religious texts to benefit the unborn child.

The Mahabharata is an ancient Indian epic that has been passed down through generations. It is a vast and complex work, consisting of over 100,000 couplets, and is believed to have been written around 400 BCE. The epic is a rich source of mythology, history, and philosophy, and has had a significant impact on Indian culture and society.

The story of Lord Krishna telling the story of chakravyuh when Subhadra is pregnant is a popular myth that has been passed down through generations. According to the myth, when Subhadra was pregnant with Abhimanyu, her brother-in-law Lord Krishna told her the story of how to enter the Chakravyuh, a complex military formation. It is believed that Abhimanyu, who was born with the knowledge of how to enter the Chakravyuh, was able to enter and break the formation during the Mahabharata war, leading to a significant victory for the Pandavas.

The historical context of this myth is rooted in the ancient Indian belief in the power of storytelling. Stories and myths were considered an important way of passing down knowledge and wisdom from one generation to the next. The Mahabharata, with its rich tapestry of stories and myths, was an important source of knowledge and wisdom for ancient Indians.

In addition, the myth also reflects the importance given to warfare and military strategy in ancient India. Military prowess was considered an essential quality for rulers and leaders, and the ability to break complex military formations was seen as a sign of great skill and intelligence. The story of Abhimanyu, who was born with the knowledge of how to enter the Chakravyuh, is an example of how important military knowledge was in ancient India.

Overall, the historical context of this myth reflects the importance given to storytelling, knowledge, and military strategy in ancient India. The myth continues to be popular today and is often cited as an example of the power of prenatal education and the transmission of knowledge from one generation to the next.

C. Scientific evidence debunking the myth

Unfortunately, there is no scientific evidence to debunk or prove the myth that Lord Krishna's story about the chakravyuh during Subhadra's pregnancy has any impact on the fetus. However, it is important to note that this story is a mythological tale and should not be taken as a medical or scientific fact.

In modern times, it is important to rely on evidence-based scientific research and medical advice to ensure the health and well-being of both the mother and the fetus during pregnancy. Relying on ancient tales or myths to guide medical decisions can be dangerous and lead to harmful consequences.

It is also worth noting that the cultural and spiritual significance of myths and ancient tales should not be dismissed or disregarded. Such stories can hold deep meaning and significance in various cultures and religions, and can offer valuable insights into the beliefs and values of a particular community. However, when it comes to matters of health and medical decisions, it is important to rely on factual and scientific information.

Overall, while the story of Lord Krishna and Subhadra may hold cultural and spiritual significance, there is no scientific evidence to support the notion that it has any impact on the fetus during pregnancy. As such, it is important to prioritize evidence-based medical care during pregnancy and consult with trained medical professionals for any questions or concerns.

D. Consequences of the myth

The belief that Garbh Sanskar can enhance the intelligence and skills of the fetus can lead to
Unnecessary stress and anxiety for expectant mothers. It can also lead to the promotion of unproven and potentially harmful practices and rituals. In some cases, it may lead to neglect of scientifically proven methods of prenatal care and development.

Additionally, the promotion of such myths can have negative consequences for women and girls, who may be forced to adhere to strict rituals and practices during pregnancy, limiting their freedom and autonomy. The perpetuation of myths like this can also reinforce harmful gender norms and stereotypes, suggesting that women's primary role is to bear and raise children.

XII. CONCLUSION

Garbh Sanskar, a concept rooted in ancient Indian traditions, is often believed to have the ability to influence the physical, mental, and emotional development of a fetus. This book aims to debunk seven prevalent myths surrounding Garbh Sanskar through scientific evidence and historical context.

The first myth, that Garbh Sanskar ensures the birth of a male child, has no scientific basis and only serves to perpetuate patriarchal attitudes. The second myth, that Garbh Sanskar can cure genetic disorders in the fetus, ignores the complex nature of genetic diseases and the limitations of Garbh Sanskar practices. The third myth, that Garbh Sanskar can increase the intelligence of the fetus, has no scientific evidence to support it and places undue pressure on expecting parents.

The fourth myth, that Garbh Sanskar can influence the physical appearance of the child, has no scientific basis and disregards the role of genetics in determining physical traits. The fifth myth, that Garbh Sanskar involves specific rituals and practices, has been influenced by commercialization and is often marketed as a product rather than a holistic approach to prenatal care.

The sixth myth, that solar and lunar eclipses affect the fetus during Garbh Sanskar, is rooted in superstition and has no scientific evidence to support it. Finally, the seventh myth, that Lord Krishna's story of chakravyuh in the Mahabharat is a reference to Garbh Sanskar, has been misinterpreted and taken out of context.

This book has several implications for society. Firstly, it highlights the importance of separating myth from reality and relying on scientific evidence when making decisions about prenatal care. The perpetuation of these myths can have harmful consequences for expecting parents, including increased stress and anxiety.

Secondly, it emphasizes the need for education and awareness about prenatal care practices that are supported by scientific evidence. This includes the importance of a balanced diet, exercise, and regular prenatal check-ups.

Lastly, it underscores the danger of commercialization and profit-driven approaches to prenatal care. The market for Garbh Sanskar products and services is often driven by misinformation and superstition, rather than evidence-based practices that promote the health and well-being of expecting mothers and their fetuses.

The prevalence of these myths surrounding Garbh Sanskar has significant implications for Indian society. It perpetuates the idea that a woman's worth is primarily tied to her ability to bear and raise healthy, intelligent, and physically attractive children. This reinforces gender stereotypes and can lead to discrimination against women who are unable to conceive or bear healthy children.

Furthermore, the promotion of these myths by self-proclaimed practitioners of Garbh Sanskar can lead to exploitation of vulnerable pregnant women and their families who are desperate to ensure the best outcomes for their children. These practitioners often charge exorbitant fees and promote unscientific practices, which can be harmful to both the mother and the fetus.

C. Recommendations for future research and practice:

To combat these myths, it is essential to promote evidence-based practices during pregnancy and childbirth. This requires a concerted effort from medical professionals, policymakers, and the public to promote scientific knowledge and debunk unfounded beliefs.

Research into the effects of maternal health and nutrition, as well as prenatal care and education, can help to identify evidence-based interventions to promote healthy pregnancies and positive birth outcomes. This research can also inform the development of culturally appropriate interventions that respect the cultural beliefs and practices of diverse communities.

Medical professionals must be trained to provide evidence-based care during pregnancy and childbirth and to engage in respectful communication with patients to address their concerns and questions. This includes working with patients to dispel myths and providing accurate information to promote informed decision-making.

Finally, it is important to engage with the public and promote critical thinking around beliefs and practices related to Garbh Sanskar. This can be done through community-based education programs, social media campaigns, and other forms of outreach. By promoting evidence-based practices and debunking myths, we can ensure that all pregnant women have access to the care and support they need to ensure the best outcomes for themselves and their children.

In conclusion, the myths surrounding Garbh Sanskar highlight the importance of promoting evidence-based practices during pregnancy and childbirth. By doing so, we can ensure that all pregnant women have access to the care and support they need to promote healthy pregnancies and positive birth outcomes. We must work together to dispel unfounded beliefs and promote critical thinking to ensure that women and their families are not exploited by unscrupulous practitioners.

And also, the seven myths surrounding Garbh Sanskar are prevalent in Indian society and perpetuate harmful attitudes and practices. It is crucial to separate fact from fiction and rely on scientific evidence when making decisions about prenatal care. The goal of prenatal care should be to promote the health and well-being of both the expecting mother and the fetus, rather than perpetuating harmful myths and commercialized practices. By debunking these myths and promoting evidence-based approaches to prenatal care, we can create a healthier and more informed society.

XIII. MYTHS OF GARBH SANSKAR AROUND THE WORLD

Exploring the myths of Garbh Sanskar takes us on a global journey, unveiling how different cultures and countries weave their own narratives around the concept of nurturing the unborn child. These myths, though diverse, reflect the universal human desire for a healthy, happy, and prosperous next generation.

In China, the ancient practice of "Zuo Yue Zi" involves specific rituals and dietary restrictions during the postpartum period, aiming to promote the health of both the mother and the newborn. The belief is deeply rooted in the idea that the well-being of the mother influences the child's health and future.

Across the ocean in Africa, various communities hold diverse beliefs about prenatal care. In some tribes, specific rituals and ceremonies are performed to protect the unborn child from negative energies, ensuring a smooth transition into the world.

In South America, indigenous cultures have their own unique practices. For instance, the Quechua people in Peru believe in the importance of maintaining a positive emotional environment during pregnancy, emphasizing the impact of a mother's emotions on the child.

In the Western world, though practices may differ, there's a growing interest in holistic approaches to prenatal care. From prenatal yoga to mindfulness practices, there's an acknowledgment of the mind-body connection during pregnancy.

While these practices vary, the common thread lies in the belief that the environment surrounding the mother, both physical and emotional, can influence the well-being of the unborn child. The power of cultural beliefs in shaping these practices transcends borders, reflecting the universal human experience of anticipating and welcoming new life.

It's crucial to recognize that these practices, though rooted in cultural wisdom, sometimes intertwine with myths. In each culture, there may be beliefs about the gender of the child, the influence of celestial events, or specific rituals that impact the child's future. As we unravel these global myths, it becomes apparent that, irrespective of cultural differences, the essence of Garbh Sanskar revolves around a shared desire for a healthy and prosperous next generation.

Understanding these diverse myths offers a broader perspective on the universal human experience of preparing for parenthood. As we navigate through the varied tapestry of beliefs, we recognize that the journey of Garbh Sanskar transcends borders, uniting humanity in the shared aspiration for the well-being and success of future generations.

XIV. LAB TESTS: DONE TO ASSESS THE HEALTH OF THE DEVELOPING BABY DURING PREGNANCY.

There are several prenatal tests that can be done to assess the health of the developing baby during pregnancy. The specific tests recommended may vary depending on the individual circumstances of the pregnancy, but some common prenatal tests include:

1.   Ultrasound: This is a non-invasive imaging test that uses high-frequency sound waves to create images of the developing fetus. Ultrasound can be used to check the baby's growth and development, assess the placenta and amniotic fluid, and detect any abnormalities or defects.

2.   Maternal blood tests: Blood tests can be used to measure various markers and hormones in the mother's blood that can indicate potential health issues in the developing baby. Examples include the quad screen, which measures levels of four different substances in the mother's blood to screen for certain chromosomal abnormalities, and the glucose tolerance test, which checks for gestational diabetes.

3.   Amniocentesis: This is an invasive test that involves taking a sample of amniotic fluid from around the developing fetus. Amniocentesis can be used to diagnose certain genetic disorders, chromosomal abnormalities, and neural tube defects.

4.   Non-invasive prenatal testing (NIPT): This is a newer type of prenatal test that can be done using a sample of the mother's blood. NIPT is used to screen for certain chromosomal abnormalities and can be done as early as 10 weeks of pregnancy.

5.	Fetal echocardiography: This is a specialized type of ultrasound that focuses on the baby's heart. Fetal echocardiography can be used to detect heart defects and other issues with the baby's cardiovascular system.

6.	Non-stress test: This is a test that measures the baby's heart rate in response to fetal movement. Non-stress testing can be used to assess fetal well-being and detect any signs of distress.

These are just a few examples of the many prenatal tests that can be done to assess the health of the developing baby during pregnancy. Expectant parents should consult with a qualified healthcare professional, such as a doctor or midwife, to determine which tests are appropriate for their individual circumstances.

XV. A NEW CHAPTER BEGINS: WELCOMING BABY KARTIK

Our hearts swelled with love and pride as we welcomed our bundle of joy, a baby boy. While we had secretly hoped for a baby girl, the universe had different plans for us, and we were blessed with a son – perfect in every way. His tiny fingers and tufts of soft hair held a magic that filled our home with warmth and laughter.

We named him Kartik, a name deeply rooted in our Hindu culture, symbolizing strength and virtue. It was a name that carried the weight of tradition, a legacy we hoped our little one would carry forward.

Kartik, our tiny blessing, became the focal point of our dreams. As parents, we aspired for him to grow into a rich and successful entrepreneur, a beacon of success and prosperity. Every coo, every smile, and every tiny milestone marked the beginning of a journey we eagerly anticipated – a journey of nurturing, guiding, and watching our son flourish.

In the midst of the celebrations, the joy extended beyond our little one to my wife. She emerged from the journey of pregnancy healthy, happy, and fine. The resilience she displayed, the sacrifices she made, and the love she poured into our family were all reflected in her glowing well-being.

As we basked in the glow of our newfound parenthood, we were reminded that this was not just the end of one story but the commencement of another. Our home was filled with the sweet melody of a baby's laughter, and our hearts overflowed with gratitude for the blessings that had graced our lives. With Baby Kartik in our arms, we eagerly embarked on this new chapter, ready to embrace the adventures and challenges that parenthood would undoubtedly bring.